BEHIND THE DIET

INTEGRATIVE NUTRITION STRATEGIES FOR CELIAC DISEASE, IBS, AND FUNCTIONAL GUT CONDITIONS

Jessica Martinez, RDN

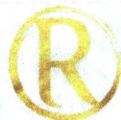

RITZ
BOOKS

Behind the Diet: Integrative Nutrition Strategies for Celiac Disease, IBS, and Functional Gut Conditions

by Jessica Martinez, RDN

Copyright © 2025 Jessica Martinez

Paperback ISBN: 978-1-960460-35-6
Kindle ISBN: 978-1-960460-36-3

Cover Design & Manuscript Layout by Steph Ritz
Published by Ritz Books

RitzBooks.com
STORIES THAT CHANGE THE WORLD
PUBLISHING FOR VISIONARY LEADERS

Please visit
http://www.stephritz.com/
to learn more.

Or email Steph@StephRitz.com
to get started today.

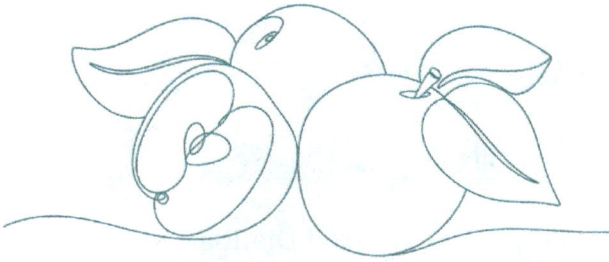

Dedication

To those who stood by me through the most challenging parts of my health and academic journey—thank you.

To my parents and sister, your unwavering belief in my vision and purpose gave me the strength to keep going and the courage to pave a path for others still searching for answers.

I also acknowledge the difficult moments, the doubt, and the absence of support. Without that adversity, I may never have learned to quiet the noise, trust my voice, and refine my skills with greater purpose.

Table of Contents

Glossary of Acronyms

CD – Celiac Disease

A chronic autoimmune condition in which ingestion of gluten leads to damage in the small intestine.

FODMAPs – Fermentable Oligosaccharides, Disaccharides, Monosaccharides, and Polyols
A group of short-chain carbohydrates that are poorly absorbed in the gut and can trigger gastrointestinal symptoms.

GF – Gluten-Free
Refers to a diet or product that excludes gluten, a protein found in wheat, barley, and rye.

IBS – Irritable Bowel Syndrome

A functional gastrointestinal disorder marked by abdominal pain, bloating, and altered bowel habits, often influenced by diet and stress.

NCGS – Non-Celiac Gluten Sensitivity

A condition where individuals experience symptoms like those of Celiac Disease when consuming gluten, but without the autoimmune response or intestinal damage.

RDN – Registered Dietitian Nutritionist

A health professional specialized in nutrition and dietetics, qualified to offer dietary guidance and counseling.

SCFAs – Short-Chain Fatty Acids:

Beneficial fatty acids produced by the fermentation of dietary fiber in the colon, important for gut health and inflammation regulation.

SIBO – Small Intestinal Bacterial Overgrowth
A condition characterized by an excessive growth of bacteria in the small intestine, leading to symptoms like bloating, gas, and diarrhea.

SMASH – Salmon, Mackerel, Anchovies, Sardines, Herring
An acronym for fatty fish high in omega-3 fatty acids, recommended for their anti-inflammatory properties.

Introduction

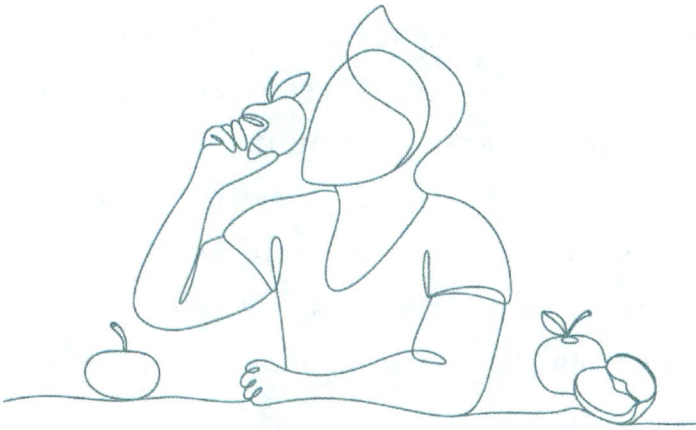

Why This Book Exists

Navigating digestive symptoms can feel like trying to solve a puzzle without all the pieces. For many, simply being told to "go gluten-free" (GF) is presented as the cure-all solution. But what happens when symptoms **persist despite removing gluten**, or a diagnosis of "just Irritable Bowel Syndrome (IBS)" without answers or direction?

This book was developed to bridge the gap between diagnosis, daily life, and effective nutrition care. Whether supporting individuals with Celiac Disease (CD), ongoing unexplained symptoms, or a generalized IBS diagnosis. This reference guide offers clarity, clinical context, and compassionate support—grounded in evidence, not online misinformation. More than a set of dietary rules, it serves as a tool to help patients rebuild trust in their bodies and regain confidence in their food choices through practical, sustainable strategies.

A Note from a Registered Dietitian Nutritionist Living with Celiac Disease

I didn't write this book just as a Registered Dietitian Nutritionist (RDN)—I wrote it as someone who has lived through the confusion, fear, and exhaustion of undiagnosed Celiac Disease. Before I ever learned about gut health professionally, I spent nearly a decade bouncing between doctors, eliminating foods, and second-guessing every bite I ate.

When I was finally diagnosed, it wasn't the end of the story—it was the beginning of a new one filled with questions no one had prepared me to answer: *Why do I still feel sick? What else could be going on? How do I live a full life without fear of food?*

This book was created for anyone who wants to deepen their understanding of gastrointestinal conditions and better support their patients through that same uncertainty.

Managing GI disorders is rarely straightforward—it's a complex process that often requires collaboration across disciplines. By integrating medical nutrition therapy with a broader clinical perspective, dietitians can play a vital role in helping individuals navigate their symptoms with clarity, compassion, and confidence.

Clinical Application: Supporting Diagnosed Digestive Conditions

Patient or client:

- Has been **diagnosed with Celiac Disease (CD)**, but continues to experience symptoms despite following a gluten-free (GF) diet

- Suspects gluten is causing issues but hasn't received a clear diagnosis

- Has been labeled with **IBS** without guidance or instructions on how to manage the condition.

- Is overwhelmed by conflicting wellness messages about low FODMAP, dairy-free, Small Intestinal Bacterial Overgrowth (SIBO) protocols, etc.

- Wants a sustainable approach to digestive health that prioritizes

function, flexibility, and mental well-being

This book serves as a clinically relevant tool for supporting individuals across the spectrum of gluten-related and functional gastrointestinal disorders-whether newly diagnosed, long-term adherence to a gluten-free diet, or those with unresolved symptoms. It provides evidence-based frameworks and therapeutic strategies that emphasize nutrition adequacy, symptom management, and patient-centered care, while avoiding fear-based or unnecessarily restrictive interventions.

Part I:

Understanding Symptoms

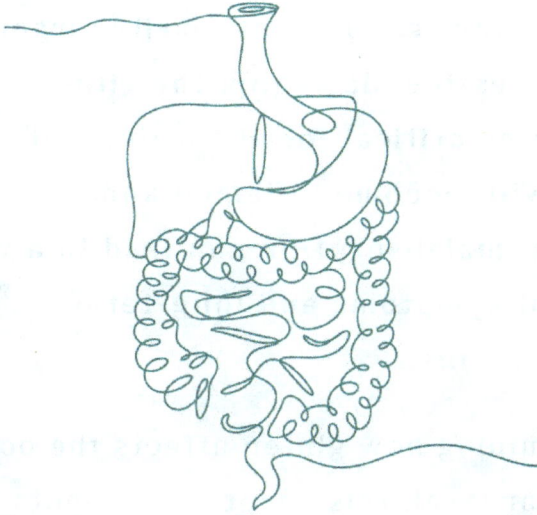

How Celiac Disease affects the body beyond the surface-level understanding of gluten avoidance

Celiac Disease is a medically complex autoimmune disease that extends far beyond the popular notion of avoiding gluten. This chapter introduces the condition by clarifying that it is not a simple intolerance, but a chronic immune reaction triggered by gluten ingestion in genetically predisposed individuals.

The **immune response primarily targets the small intestine, damaging the villi—small structures critical for absorbing nutrients. As the villi become inflamed and atrophied, nutrient malabsorption can lead to a wide range of symptoms and long-term complications.**

By examining how gluten affects the body at a cellular level, this chapter highlights the importance of timely diagnosis, strict dietary adherence, and ongoing medical oversight to support whole-body health in those with Celiac Disease.

Chapter 1:
Celiac Disease –
More Than Just a Gluten-Free Diet

Celiac Disease is often misunderstood as a simple food intolerance. In reality, it is a **chronic autoimmune disease**—meaning the body's immune system mistakenly attacks its own tissues in response to gluten, a protein found in wheat, barley, and rye. This reaction is **not limited to the digestive tract**. Instead, it causes widespread damage throughout the body, especially if left undiagnosed or mismanaged.

What Happens in the Body?

The primary site of damage is the **small intestine,** where tiny finger-like projections called **villi** help absorb nutrients from food. In people with Celiac Disease, consuming gluten leads to **inflammation and destruction** of these villi, a process known as **villous atrophy**. Without healthy villi, the body cannot absorb vitamins, minerals, and other nutrients properly.

As a result, people with Celiac Disease may develop:

- **Iron deficiency anemia** (from poor iron absorption)
- **Osteoporosis** or weakened bones (from low calcium and Vitamin D)
- **Fatigue**, brain fog, and neurological symptoms
- **Fertility challenges** or menstrual irregularities
- **Skin disorders**, like dermatitis herpetiformis (an itchy, blistering rash)

This means that **Celiac Disease is not just about stomach issues**. Even without diarrhea or bloating, damage can still occur silently over time.

Understanding the Digestive Tract: A Brief Overview

Digestive health is dependent on a **complex process** that starts in the mouth and ends in the intestines. At every step, specific **enzymes** in the mouth and stomach break food down into usable nutrients.

Human Digestive System

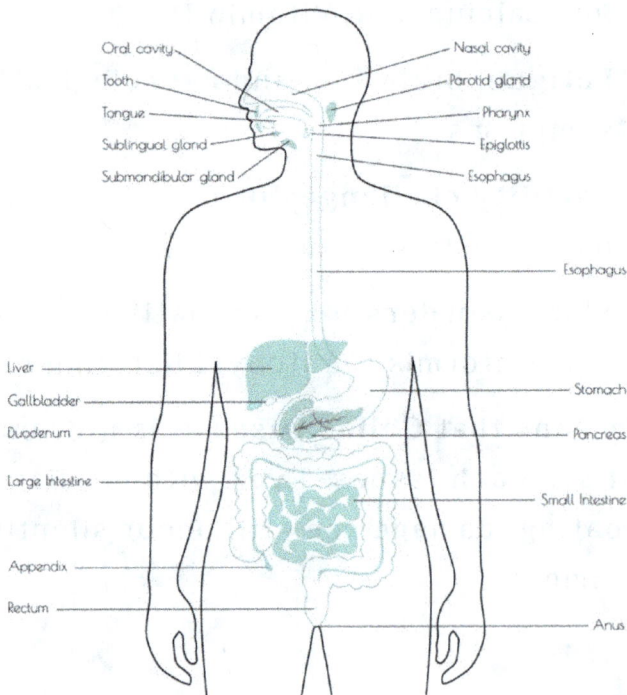

Oral cavity	Nasal cavity
Tooth	Parotid gland
Tongue	Pharynx
Sublingual gland	Epiglottis
Submandibular gland	Esophagus
	Esophagus
Liver	Stomach
Gallbladder	Pancreas
Duodenum	
Large Intestine	Small Intestine
Appendix	
Rectum	Anus

Step 1: Mouth – Where Digestion Begins

Digestion starts when food enters the mouth. This is not just about chewing, **enzymes in the saliva** begin to catabolize food.

- **Salivary amylase**: Begins breaking down starches into sugars (Freitas et al., 2018)
- **Lingual lipase**: Starts breaking down fats (Armand, 2007)

Chewing well and allowing saliva to mix with food improves the catabolic process before it reaches the stomach.

Step 2: Stomach – Breaking Down Proteins

In the stomach, food mixes with powerful acids and enzymes that begin the breakdown process:

- **Pepsin** (activated from pepsinogen by stomach acid): Begins breaking down proteins into smaller chains.
- **Gastric lipase**: Helps break down fats.

- **Hydrochloric acid (HCl)**: Unfolds proteins and kills harmful microbes that may be found in the food.

The stomach's role is mostly about breaking food apart, not absorbing nutrients. Once food is processed into a semi-liquid form called chyme, it moves into the small intestine—the main hub for absorption.

SMALL INTESTINE

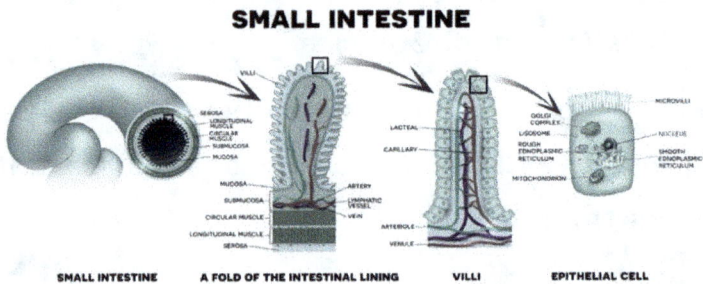

| SMALL INTESTINE | A FOLD OF THE INTESTINAL LINING | VILLI | EPITHELIAL CELL |

Step 3: Small Intestine – The Main Site of Absorption

The small intestine is a long, coiled tube divided into three parts:

- **Duodenum**
- **Jejunum**
- **Ileum**

Each section plays a unique role in absorbing nutrients that the body needs.

Duodenum – Absorbs Most Minerals

This first section connects directly to the stomach and receives digestive juices from the pancreas and bile from the liver. These digestive juices help neutralize stomach acid and continue catabolizing food.

Main nutrients absorbed here:

- **Iron** – Carries oxygen in the blood
- **Calcium** – Builds strong bones and supports nerve and muscle function
- **Magnesium** and **Zinc** – Support immune function and many enzymatic processes
- **Vitamin A** – Supports vision and immune function

The duodenum is especially important for mineral absorption, thanks to its acidic-to-alkaline environment that helps make minerals easier to absorb.

Jejunum – Absorbs Water-Soluble Vitamins and Macronutrients

The jejunum is the middle section and does most of the heavy lifting when it comes to nutrient absorption.

Key nutrients absorbed here:

- *Water-soluble vitamins, including:*

  - *Vitamin C – Helps with healing and immune defense*

  - *B-complex vitamins (B1, B2, B3, B5, B6, biotin, folate) – Involved in energy production, nerve health, and making red blood cells*

- *Carbohydrates – Absorbed as simple sugars*

- *Proteins – Absorbed as amino acids*

Water-soluble vitamins don't need fat to be absorbed and go straight into the bloodstream after passing through the lining of the jejunum.

Ileum – Absorbs Fat-Soluble Vitamins and Bile

Salts

The ileum is the last section of the small intestine, and although most nutrients have already been absorbed, it plays a vital role in picking up what's left.

- **Nutrients absorbed in the ileum:**
  - *Fat-soluble vitamins, including:*
    - *Vitamin D – Helps absorb calcium for bones*
    - *Vitamin E – Acts as an antioxidant*
    - *Vitamin K – Supports blood clotting*
  - *Vitamin B12 – Essential for nerves and red blood cell production*
  - *Bile salts – Reabsorbed here and sent back to the liver to be reused*

What Are Bile Salts and Why Are They Important?

Bile salts are made in the liver and stored in the gallbladder. When food is eaten that contain fat, bile salts are released into the duodenum to help break that fat into smaller droplets—a process called **emulsification**.

- **Think of bile salts like dish soap**: They break up fat so enzymes can work more effectively.

- After doing their job, **bile salts are reabsorbed in the ileum** and recycled back to the liver. This process is called **enterohepatic circulation**.

Key Takeaways

Digestion starts in the mouth and involves a series of enzymes that break food into smaller pieces the body can use.

The stomach initiates protein and fat digestion but doesn't absorb nutrients.

The small intestine—especially the brush border of the duodenum, jejunum, and ileum—is the main site for nutrient absorption.

The duodenum absorbs key minerals like iron and calcium.

The jejunum is where most water-soluble vitamins and nutrients like carbs and protein are absorbed.

The ileum handles most fat-soluble vitamins, Vitamin B12, and bile salts.

In Celiac Disease, the body attacks the small intestine after gluten is consumed, damaging the villi and preventing proper nutrient absorption.

If the villi (tiny fingerlike projections) in the small intestine are damaged—such as in Celiac Disease—nutrient absorption is severely affected, no matter how healthy someone eats.

Without healthy villi and microvilli, the body struggles to absorb essential nutrients—even if the diet is balanced.

Why Testing Before Starting a Gluten-Free Diet Matters

A common mistake is to start a gluten-free diet prior to getting tested for Celiac Disease, gluten intolerance, or gluten allergy. This may lead to **false-negative test results and make future diagnosis difficult**. CD testing is used to identify the immune system's reaction to gluten, so **gluten must be actively consume**d for accurate results.

Standard testing includes blood tests such as anti-TTG IgA (a marker of autoimmune activity). If the blood test is positive, a biopsy of the duodenum is used to confirm damage.

Additionally, **IgA deficiency**—a condition that affects about 2-3% of CD patients—can lead to misleading results. In such cases, **alternative markers like DGP** or **IgG-based tests** may be used (Husby et al., 2020).

Unfortunately, many individuals are **misdiagnosed with Irritable Bowel Syndrome (IBS)** before being screened for Celiac Disease. A UK study found that up to **1 in 5 people with Celiac Disease remain undiagnosed**, often for years (Shahbazkhani et al., 2003).

The Gluten-Free Diet Isn't Always Enough

While the only current treatment for Celiac Disease is strict, lifelong adherence to avoiding **gluten, studies show that up to 30% of patients continue to experience symptoms** despite following the diet carefully (Roos et al., 2019).

Reasons may include:

- Hidden gluten exposure
- Co-existing conditions (e.g., lactose intolerance, IBS)
- Nutrient deficiencies that linger due to prior damage
- Ongoing intestinal inflammation

Managing Celiac Disease requires more than label-reading. It involves **strategic nutrition support**, follow-up testing, and sometimes, **gut protocols** supervised by healthcare professionals.

Key Takeaways

Celiac Disease is a systemic condition—it affects far more than digestion.

Lifelong gluten avoidance is critical, but not always enough for full recovery.

Testing must occur while gluten is still in the diet to avoid false negatives.

Proper diagnosis and long-term follow-up are essential to prevent complications and ensure optimal health.

Chapter 2:
When Symptoms Don't Stop — Untangling IBS, Celiac Disease, and Non-Celiac Gluten Sensitivity

Celiac Disease is a serious autoimmune disease—not simply a digestive issue—and that it requires more than removing gluten. But what if symptoms persist, or a patient has already tried a GF diet and isn't getting better? What if the doctor diagnosed "IBS" without much explanation?

This chapter dives into the **gray zones of gut health**, where symptoms blur together and misdiagnoses are common. Three conditions in particular—**Celiac Disease (CD)**, **Irritable Bowel Syndrome (IBS)**, and **Non-Celiac Gluten Sensitivity (NCGS)**—can all cause similar distress but stem from **entirely**

different mechanisms. Understanding these differences is crucial, not only for effective treatment, but also for quality of life.

Different Roots, Same Symptoms

Bloating, gas, cramps, unpredictable bowel habits—these symptoms are common across all three conditions. What sets them apart is **what's happening beneath the surface**:

- **Celiac Disease** is an **autoimmune reaction** to gluten that causes measurable damage to the small intestine.

- **IBS** is a **functional gut disorder**, meaning the symptoms are real but arise from how the gut behaves—not from damage or inflammation.

- **NCGS** involves gluten-like symptoms, **but without immune system involvement or visible intestinal damage**.

This overlap can be confusing. Someone might remove gluten, feel better, and assume they have Celiac Disease—when they may actually have IBS or NCGS. Or worse, someone with true Celiac Disease might be told it's "just IBS" and go years without the correct diagnosis.

IBS: A Gut That's Out of Sync

Irritable Bowel Syndrome is one of the most common gastrointestinal conditions, affecting around **10–15% of people globally**. It's defined by the **Rome IV Criteria**, which include:

- Recurring abdominal discomfort: pain occurring at least one day per week over the past 3 months.

- Accompanied by at least two of the following features:
  - Pain is linked to bowel movements
  - Noticeable by changes in how often stools occur

♦ Alteration in stool appearance or texture

These symptoms should have first appeared within the last 6 months.

What makes IBS so difficult is that there is **no test for it**. Instead, it's diagnosed by ruling out other conditions. The exact causes of IBS vary, but common contributors include:

- **Gut-brain axis disruption** (the communication loop between the brain and GI tract)

- **Abnormal motility** (food moves too fast or too slow)

- **Food triggers**, especially **FODMAPs** (a group of fermentable carbs that feed gas-producing gut bacteria)

- **Stress**, **trauma**, or **anxiety**, which can heighten gut sensitivity

Importantly, **IBS doesn't cause permanent damage**, but it can severely affect quality of life if not managed appropriately.

Non-Celiac Gluten Sensitivity: The Middle Ground

NCGS is a condition where individuals experience digestive or systemic symptoms—such as bloating, fatigue, brain fog, or joint pain—after eating gluten, but **do not test positive for Celiac Disease and do not show intestinal damage** in their biopsy.

In some studies, individuals with NCGS report feeling better on a GF diet—but when being blinded to what they're eating, some **reacted more strongly to FODMAPs (like fructans) than to gluten itself** (Biesiekierski et al., 2013). This raises the question: Is gluten the true trigger, or is it a scapegoat?

Still, NCGS is real. It's not psychosomatic. But it's a **diagnosis of exclusion**, meaning it should only be considered after other conditions—including Celiac Disease and/or a wheat allergy—have been ruled out through testing.

How Misdiagnosis Happens

The overlap in symptoms leads to **a high rate of diagnostic error**, especially when individuals self-eliminate gluten before testing. In fact, research shows that **Celiac Disease is four times more likely to be found in people originally diagnosed with IBS** than in the general population (Ford et al., 2024).

Mislabeling someone with IBS when they have Celiac Disease can delay necessary treatment and increase the risk of complications like malnutrition, osteoporosis, and neurological problems. On the other hand, labeling someone with CD or gluten sensitivity when they have IBS may lead them to unnecessarily restrict their diet, potentially worsening nutrient intake and social distress.

Why Testing — and Timing — Matters

If patients or clients continue with chronic digestive symptoms—bloating, cramping, irregular bowel movements, or unexplained fatigue—it's natural to wonder whether gluten may be the cause. Many people experiment by removing gluten from their diets, hoping to feel better. While this might offer temporary relief, eliminating gluten **before proper testing can complicate or even prevent an accurate diagnosis** of CD or NCGS.

To understand why timing is crucial, it helps to look at how CD is diagnosed—and why the presence of gluten in an individual's diet is essential for this process.

Celiac Disease: Diagnosis Depends on an Active Immune Response

Celiac Disease is diagnosed using a **two-step approach**:

1. Serologic Testing

The most used test is **anti-tissue transglutaminase IgA (anti-tTG IgA)**. This test looks for antibodies produced by the immune system in response to gluten exposure in genetically predisposed individuals. Genetic markers are HLA-DQ2 and HLA-DQ8, which we will discuss in the next chapter.

Other blood tests may include:

- Total serum IgA (to rule out IgA deficiency, which affects test accuracy)

- Deamidated gliadin peptide (DGP) IgG, especially in IgA-deficient patients

- Endomysial antibody (EMA), which is highly specific but less commonly used due to cost and complexity

2. **Intestinal Biopsy**
   If blood tests are positive, the next step is usually a biopsy of the small intestine via upper endoscopy. This allows for microscopic evaluation of the intestinal

lining to detect **villous atrophy**, the hallmark of CD.

Biopsy results are graded using the **Marsh-Oberhuber classification**, which ranges from Marsh 0 (normal mucosa) to Marsh lllc (complete villous flattening) (Husby et al., 2020).

But here's the catch: **these antibodies and intestinal changes only occur in response to gluten exposure**. If an individual has been off gluten for several weeks or months, the immune system may no longer be actively reacting—resulting in a **false-negative result**, even if they do have Celiac Disease.

Chapter 3:
The Diagnostic Dilemma

However, many individuals begin a GF diet prior to completing appropriate diagnostic testing, often out of desperation to relieve symptoms or based on non-medical advice. **These premature dietary changes can significantly compromise the diagnostic process.** Celiac Disease serologic testing— most notably the tissue transglutaminase IgA (tTG-IgA) and endomysial antibody (EMA) tests—requires active gluten consumption to detect the autoimmune response characteristics of the disease. Once gluten is eliminated from the diet, these antibodies may normalize, leading to **false-negative results**, even in individuals with true Celiac Disease (Rubio-Tapia et al., 2013).

Additionally, approximately **2–3% of individuals with Celiac Disease have selective IgA deficiency**, one of the most common primary immunodeficiencies. In these cases, IgA-based tests such as tTG-IgA may also yield false-negative results despite active disease. To avoid misdiagnosis, **total serum IgA should be measured concurrently**, and if deficiency is detected, **IgG-based assays** (e.g., deamidated gliadin peptide IgG or tTG-IgG) must be used instead (Hill et al., 2016).

To further clarify ambiguous or inconclusive cases—particularly when patients are already gluten-free—**HLA-DQ2** and **HLA-DQ8 genetic testing** can be a valuable tool. While not diagnostic on their own, the absence of both alleles **virtually excludes Celiac Disease.** Conversely, a positive result indicates genetic susceptibility but requires gluten reintroduction and formal testing to confirm active disease. This step is essential because individuals who are genetically predisposed but remain undiagnosed and untreated may continue to suffer from subtle intestinal damage. They are at elevated risk for long-term complications, including **osteoporosis, infertility, iron-deficiency anemia**, and **other autoimmune conditions** (Lebwohl et al., 2018).

When left untreated or improperly managed, Celiac Disease causes **immune-mediated destruction of the small intestinal villi**, particularly in the duodenum and proximal jejunum—the primary sites of **nutrient absorption**. As villous atrophy progresses, the body's ability to absorb **iron, folate, calcium, magnesium, fat-soluble vitamins (A, D, E, K)**, and **Vitamin B12** becomes impaired. This can lead to multisystemic manifestations such as **fatigue, neurologic symptoms, osteopenia/osteoporosis, menstrual irregularities**, and **delayed growth in children** (Green & Cellier, 2007). Persistent inflammation in the small intestine may also increase the risk of more severe complications, including **intestinal lymphoma** or **refractory Celiac Disease** in rare cases.

Key Clinical Implications:

- Always test **before** initiating a gluten-free diet to ensure accurate diagnosis and long-term monitoring.

- Assess total serum IgA to identify individuals who may require alternative testing.

- Use HLA typing when diagnosis is unclear, especially if the patient has already eliminated gluten or presents with atypical symptoms.

- Emphasize that Celiac Disease is not simply a digestive disorder—it is a systemic autoimmune condition requiring lifelong management and routine surveillance.

Healthcare providers must be vigilant in assessing patients' dietary habits and consider genetic testing or a supervised gluten challenge when necessary.

Key Takeaways:

Early dietary changes can complicate diagnosis.

Alternative testing may be required for accurate results.

Collaboration between patient and provider is crucial.

Why Not to Go Gluten-Free Before Testing

If an individual is experiencing digestive symptoms and suspect Celiac Disease, it's very important not to start a gluten-free diet before getting tested. Here's why:

Celiac Disease is diagnosed by looking for specific antibodies in the blood and by examining the lining of the small intestine for damage. But these signs only show up **when gluten is still in the patient's diet**. Once gluten is removed, the body may stop producing the antibodies, and the intestine may start to heal — which can lead to a **false-negative test result**.

What the Research Shows

To ensure accurate Celiac Disease testing, **experts recommend consuming 1 to 3 servings of gluten-containing foods daily**— such as bread or pasta—for 6 to 8 weeks before testing. This ongoing exposure helps trigger the immune response and allows for the detection of antibodies and intestinal damage if Celiac Disease is present (Lebwohl et al., 2018).

Some recent studies suggest that shorter gluten challenges may also provoke measurable immune changes. For instance, one 2020 trial showed that **3 grams of gluten daily for just 14 days** could lead to detectable responses in individuals suspected of having Celiac Disease (Leonard et al., 2021).

Despite these findings, the current recommendation remains to **continue eating gluten** until a healthcare provider advises otherwise, to avoid false-negative results.

Removing Gluten Too Soon

If removing gluten before testing:

- Blood tests may come back normal, even if they have Celiac Disease.

- A biopsy might not show the damage because the small intestine has started to heal.

- Misdiagnosis or no diagnosis, delaying the right treatment.

This is why researchers at Columbia University and other experts emphasize: *Don't start a gluten-free diet until all testing is complete.*

What If the Tests Are Negative but Symptoms Persist?

If both serology and biopsy come back normal, yet symptoms continue, other possibilities include:

- **Non-Celiac Gluten Sensitivity (NCGS)** Diagnosis here is based on exclusion: negative Celiac Disease tests, no wheat allergy, but symptom relief with a GF diet. No specific biomarkers currently exist, which makes diagnosis more nuanced.

- **FODMAP intolerance or IBS**
  In some cases, it's not gluten but
  fructans, a FODMAP found in wheat,
  that triggers symptoms—common in
  individuals with IBS (Biesiekierski et al.,
  2013).

Why Skipping the Testing Stage Can Be Harmful

Going gluten-free before medical evaluation
might seem like a harmless step. But doing so
can lead to:

- **Missed or delayed diagnosis of Celiac Disease**, increasing the risk of long-term complications like osteoporosis, anemia, infertility, or lymphoma

- **Unnecessary dietary restrictions** if symptoms stem from another issue, such as IBS or a FODMAP intolerance

- **Increased psychological burden**, as strict dietary rules without medical clarity can lead to food fear and nutritional imbalance

Moreover, once gluten has been removed, **reintroducing it can be physically difficult,** as symptoms may return more intensely, making the gluten challenge a distressing process if not medically supervised.

Therapeutic Framework

To avoid diagnostic delays, follow this evidence-based testing approach:

1. **No removal of gluten until testing is complete**, unless medically directed.

2. **Begins with serologic screening,** particularly anti-tTG IgA and total IgA levels.

3. **Proceed with small intestine biopsy** if bloodwork is suggestive or equivocal.

4. If already GF, discuss the potential for a **gluten challenge** with physician.

5. If Celiac Disease is ruled out, but symptoms improve on a GF diet, work with a Registered Dietitian or Gastroenterologist to assess for NCGS or other intolerances.

Key Takeaways

Celiac Disease diagnosis requires active gluten exposure; otherwise, antibody levels may fall below detectable thresholds.

A gluten challenge may be needed if gluten was eliminated before testing.

Misdiagnosis or self-diagnosis can lead to unnecessary restrictions or missed treatment opportunities.

Work with a healthcare provider to ensure safe, accurate, and personalized evaluation.

Part ll:
After the Gluten-Free
Diagnosis

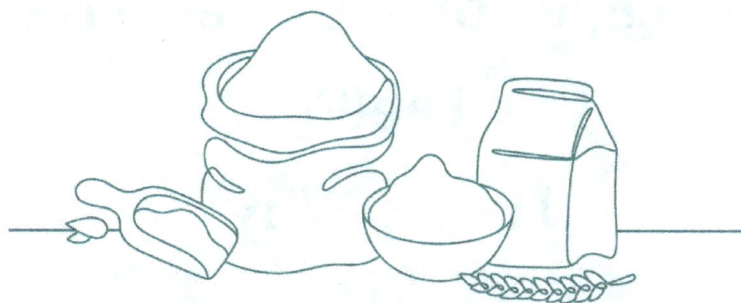

Why Symptoms May Persist Even After Cutting Out Gluten

The gluten-free diet is medically necessary for managing Celiac Disease, yet for many people, symptoms like bloating, diarrhea, or fatigue persist long after gluten has been removed. In this section, we explore hidden sources of gluten, cross-contact, other food intolerances, and micronutrient gaps that may be fueling symptoms. Even with strict adherence, the complexity of digestion and immune function means healing is not always linear.

Chapter 4:
Struggles on a Gluten-Free Diet?
Here's Why

The individual has removed gluten, reads labels, avoids wheat, barley, and rye, and checks for cross-contact. Symptoms like bloating, fatigue, or frequent trips to the bathroom—sometimes all three—can still occur despite adhering to a GF diet.

Studies show that **up to 30% of individuals with Celiac Disease continue to experience symptoms** even after eliminating gluten from their diet (Silvester et al., 2020). This chapter explores **why symptoms may persist**—and steps to take next.

1. Hidden Gluten Exposure: It's More

Common Than Most Realize

Even the tiniest amount of gluten—**as little as 10–50 mg**—can trigger symptoms and cause damage in someone with Celiac Disease. That's smaller than a breadcrumb. Despite best efforts, accidental exposure remains a frequent cause of lingering symptoms.

Common sources include:

- **Cross-contact in shared kitchens** (sponges, cutting boards, utensils, dish towels, bowels, plastic wear, self-serve food items: bulk bins, dispenser goods)

- **Restaurant meals**, even when marked "gluten-free"

- **Misleading labels** on packaged foods (e.g., "wheat free" isn't the same as certified GF)

- **Oats contaminated with wheat during processing**, unless certified GF

This is why symptom persistence **doesn't always mean the diet is failing**—it may mean an individual is unknowingly exposed to gluten in trace amounts.

2. Refractory Celiac Disease: When Symptoms Continue

In rare cases, symptoms continue despite **strict adherence** to a GF diet for more than 12 months. This may be a sign of **Refractory Celiac Disease (RCD)**—a serious condition where the immune system remains active even without gluten exposure.

RCD affects **fewer than 1–2%** of people with Celiac Disease (Lebwohl et al., 2012) and requires careful evaluation by a specialist. There are two types:

- **Type I RCD**: Abnormal immune response, but still responsive to treatment
- **Type II RCD**: Associated with abnormal immune cells and a higher risk of complications, including intestinal lymphoma

Persistent weight loss, anemia, malnutrition, or signs of nutrient deficiency despite strict dietary adherence are red flags that warrant further testing.

3. It Might Not Be (Just) Celiac Disease: Overlapping GI Conditions

Another possibility is that **Celiac Disease is not the only issue**. Several other gastrointestinal disorders can **coexist with or mimic CD symptoms**, especially if the gut hasn't fully healed.

Common overlapping conditions include:

- **IBS**: May persist after Celiac Disease diagnosis; symptoms like bloating and abdominal pain may be triggered by FODMAPs, not gluten
- **SIBO**: Excess bacteria in the small intestine causing gas, bloating, and malabsorption

- **Microscopic Colitis**: Inflammation of the colon, often causing chronic diarrhea

- **Pancreatic Insufficiency**: The pancreas fails to produce enough enzymes, impairing digestion, especially of fats

Because these conditions often overlap, **a full gastrointestinal evaluation is critical** if symptoms persist beyond the first year of a GF diet.

4. Nutrient Gaps and Fiber Deficiency: A Silent Contributor

People with Celiac Disease often adopt restrictive diets to avoid gluten, but in doing so, **many unintentionally limit fiber, B vitamins, iron**, and **other nutrients**. Inadequate intake of these nutrients can contribute to ongoing symptoms such as constipation, fatigue, or irregular stools.

In one study, individuals with Celiac Disease on a GF diet consumed **significantly less**

fiber than recommended, and many still experienced bloating and gastrointestinal discomfort (Silvester et al., 2021). This highlights the need for **balanced, whole-food-based nutrition**—not just label-reading.

Clinical Nutrition Interventions

Recovery from Celiac Disease is often **non-linear** and can take time. However, persistent symptoms deserve attention.

Actions for RDNs:

- **Conduct a comprehensive dietary assessment** to identify potential sources of hidden gluten and evaluate for micronutrient insufficiencies, particularly in fiber, B vitamins, magnesium, and iron.

- **Collaborate with the healthcare team** to recommend appropriate testing for overlapping gastrointestinal disorders (e.g., IBS, SIBO, lactose intolerance) when symptoms persist despite documented gluten-free adherence.

- **Perform a nutrient analysis** to guide individualized supplementation or dietary modifications as needed.

- **Provide ongoing education and counseling** to reinforce adherence, set realistic expectations for gut healing, and support long-term symptom monitoring and recovery.

Key Takeaways

Lingering symptoms are common and don't always mean treatment failure.

Cross-contact is one of the most common reasons for ongoing symptoms, even on a strict gluten-free diet.

Refractory Celiac Disease is rare, but serious, and requires expert evaluation.

Other GI conditions—like IBS, SIBO, and microscopic colitis—can coexist with Celiac Disease and contribute to symptoms.

Proper follow-up, medical evaluation, and nutrition support are essential for full recovery.

Chapter 5:
Beyond Gluten – Other Food Triggers to Consider

Beyond Gluten: Understanding Other Dietary Triggers in Celiac Disease and IBS

Many individuals who adopt a GF diet to manage Celiac Disease or NCGS report persistent gastrointestinal (GI) symptoms such as bloating, gas, or abdominal discomfort—even when they are strictly avoiding gluten. This lingering discomfort often leads to the question: What else might be causing these symptoms?

Recent research suggests that for some, the issue may not be gluten itself, but rather a group of poorly absorbed short-chain carbohydrates known collectively as FODMAPs—an acronym for **Fermentable Oligosaccharides, Disaccharides, Monosaccharides, and Polyols**. These compounds are naturally present in many foods. It can be difficult to digest for people with sensitive gastrointestinal tracts, such as those with CD, IBS, or SIBO (Bellini et al., 2020).

Fructans: A Type of Oligosaccharide

Fructans are chains of fructose molecules that the human body lacks the enzymes to digest. Instead, they are fermented by gut bacteria in the colon, producing gas and attracting water into the intestine, which can trigger bloating, cramping, or diarrhea.

Common Foods High in Fructans Include:

- **Wheat, barley**, and **rye** (even though gluten foods are removed, these grains still contain fructans)
- **Onions** (especially white, yellow, and red onions)
- **Garlic**

- **Leeks, shallots**, and **spring onions** (especially the white bulb portion)

- **Inulin** and **chicory root extract** (often added to "high fiber" processed foods)

Even after removing gluten, people consuming GF products that still contain these ingredients may continue to experience symptoms due to their fructan content.

Polyols: Sugar Alcohols in Fruits and Sweeteners

Polyols are sugar alcohols that are only partially absorbed in the small intestine. Like fructans, they draw water into the bowel and are fermented by gut bacteria, which can result in similar GI symptoms.

Common Polyols and Their Food Sources Include:

- **Sorbitol**: Found in apples, pears, peaches, nectarines, plums, and apricots

- **Mannitol**: Present in cauliflower, mushrooms, and snow peas

- **Xylitol**, **erythritol**, and **maltitol**: Used in sugar-free gums, candies, and some "low carb" or "keto-friendly" snacks

These compounds are often labeled as "sugar-free" or "diabetic-friendly," yet they can trigger significant discomfort in sensitive individuals.

Other Common Contributors to Persistent Symptoms

- **Lactose**: Many newly diagnosed Celiac Disease patients experience secondary lactose intolerance due to damage of the intestinal lining (brush border barrier), which affects lactase enzyme production. Until the gut heals, dairy may cause bloating, gas, or diarrhea.

- **Histamines** and **Food Additives**: Certain individuals may experience symptoms due to **histamine intolerance** or sensitivity to **food additives** like sulfites, nitrates, and benzoates, which are commonly found in processed or aged foods such as wine, cured meats, smoked fish, and some cheeses. One manifestation of histamine intolerance is a skin condition called urticaria (commonly known as hives), which appears as red, itchy welts on the skin. In some cases, dermatitis herpetiformis—a chronic, blistering rash associated specifically with Celiac Disease—may also occur if gluten exposure persists.

Key Takeaways:

A gluten-free diet alone may not resolve all digestive symptoms.

FODMAPs like fructans and polyols are frequent, overlooked triggers in both Celiac Disease and IBS populations.

Lactose intolerance and histamine sensitivity are additional contributors to ongoing symptoms.

An RDN-guided elimination and reintroduction process—such as the Low FODMAP diet—can help identify true triggers while maintaining nutritional adequacy and avoiding overly restrictive eating patterns.

Chapter 6:
Nutrition Pitfalls and Deficiencies

Are All Gluten-Free Foods Gut-Friendly? The Hidden Risks of Over-Processed GF Products

When beginning a GF diet, many people turn to packaged GF products as quick and easy substitutes for breads, cereals, baked goods, and snacks. While these items can provide short-term convenience, over-relying on them may lead to **ongoing digestive symptoms**, **nutrient gaps**, and **inflammation**—even when no gluten is present.

Why Processed GF Foods May Cause Problems

Many shelf-stable GF foods are made with **refined starches** like white rice flour, potato starch, or tapioca. These ingredients are low in fiber and protein, and they have a **high glycemic index**, which can cause blood sugar spikes and contribute to **gut and systemic inflammation** over time (Missbach et al., 2015). To make up for taste and texture, manufacturers often add **high amounts of sugar**, **sodium**, and **unhealthy fats**, which can irritate the digestive tract and worsen symptoms like bloating, gas, and cramping.

Among the health-conscious, well-educated GF consumers, many still had significant nutrient deficiencies, particularly in **magnesium**, **calcium**, **iron**, **fiber**, and **several B vitamins**. The deficiencies are partly due to avoiding naturally nutrient-rich sources like grains, legumes, dairy, and instead depending on nutrient-poor GF alternatives.

GF diets often lack critical nutrients due to limited fortification and overreliance on processed substitutes. Common deficiencies include:

- **Iron**, **Folate**, and **Vitamin B12**: Due to malabsorption or poor dietary intake.

- **Vitamin D** and **Calcium**: Important for bone health, particularly in patients with long-standing villous atrophy.

- **Magnesium** and **Zinc**: Key nutrients for gut support

Both **magnesium** and **zinc** play important roles in supporting a healthy gut—especially during times of inflammation or damage, such as with Celiac Disease or chronic digestive issues.

- **Zinc** is essential for tissue repair and helps maintain the integrity of the intestinal lining. When the gut is damaged—like in cases of leaky gut or after gluten exposure in someone with Celiac Disease—zinc supports the regeneration of the cells that line the digestive tract. It also plays a major role in immune function, helping the body fight off infections that could worsen gut inflammation.

- **Magnesium** helps relax the muscles in the digestive tract, which supports smooth bowel movements and reduces cramping. It also regulates enzymes involved in digestion and helps lower inflammation—making it easier for the gut to heal over time. Many people with GI conditions are deficient in magnesium due to poor absorption, so repleting levels can make a noticeable difference in how the gut feels and functions.

Important Note: While magnesium and zinc play valuable roles in reducing inflammation, supporting gut repair, and promoting healthy digestion, excessive intake—particularly through supplements—can lead to side effects. Zinc, when taken in high doses, may block copper absorption and weaken immune function Excessive magnesium can also cause issues, depending on the type. **Magnesium citrate** and **magnesium oxide** are more likely to cause loose stools or digestive upset, especially at higher doses. In contrast, **magnesium glycinate** is generally gentler on the digestive tract and less likely to trigger these effects.

Together, magnesium and zinc help calm inflammation, support the repair of damaged gut tissue, and keep digestion running smoothly—when used safely and appropriately.

Before adding any new supplement, it's important to consult with a healthcare provider or Registered Dietitian Nutritionist (RDN) to ensure it's appropriate for individual needs and health conditions.

The Takeaway

Ideally, a Gluten Free diet should focus on **naturally GF whole foods**—vegetables, fruits, legumes, lean proteins, nuts, seeds, and ancient grains like quinoa and millet. These foods provide essential fiber, micronutrients, and anti-inflammatory compounds that help gut repair and function at its best.

While processed GF products can be a helpful convenience—especially early in a diagnosis—they should not make up the core of an individual's daily diet. Most packaged GF foods are highly refined and low in essential nutrients, particularly **fiber, iron, zinc, magnesium, B vitamins**, and **antioxidants** (Pinto-Sánchez et al., 2018; Hallert et al., 2019). Over-reliance on these foods can slow or even reverse healing in individuals with Celiac Disease or ongoing GI symptoms.

The Hidden Problem with Processed Gluten-Free Foods

Many GF replacement products—such as GF breads, crackers, cereals, and snacks—are made with white rice flour, potato starch, or tapioca starch. While these ingredients are free of gluten, they often:

- Lack dietary fiber, which is crucial for gut motility and microbiome health
- Cause spikes in blood sugar, which may affect energy and mood
- Provide little satiety, contributing to overeating or nutrient imbalance

A study by Missbach et al. 2015 found that many GF-labeled products have **less protein and fiber**, and **more added fat**, **sugar**, and **salt** than their gluten-containing counterparts. This makes a whole-food approach essential—not just to avoid symptoms, but to restore nutritional adequacy.

True Gut Repair: What It Really Involves

Repairing the gut after years of inflammation or undiagnosed Celiac Disease is not as simple as eliminating gluten. It requires **restoring nutrient stores**, repairing intestinal lining integrity, and supporting a healthy gut microbiome.

Key components of a gut-healing plan include:

- **Whole, naturally GF foods**: Vegetables, fruits, legumes (as tolerated), GF whole grains (quinoa, buckwheat, millet), nuts, seeds, eggs, poultry, and fish. These provide **prebiotic fibers**, **antioxidants**, and **phytonutrients** that support tissue repair and microbial diversity.

- **Targeted supplementation**: Due to long-term malabsorption, individuals with CD are often deficient in **iron, Vitamin D, calcium, folate, Vitamin B12**, and **zinc**— even after beginning a GF diet (Di Sabatino et al., 2021). A healthcare provider may recommend lab testing and tailored supplements to correct these imbalances.

- **Ongoing monitoring and professional guidance**: Studies show that working with a **RDN** improves nutritional adequacy, promotes dietary variety, and reduces the risk of continued unintentional gluten exposure (Shepherd & Gibson, 2013). Even among patients who report strict adherence to the GF diet, many continue to suffer from symptoms due to FODMAP intolerance, cross-contamination, or incomplete healing of the intestinal lining.

Key Takeaways

Regular micronutrient monitoring is essential for managing long-term nutritional risks in Celiac Disease.

Strategic supplementation often supports recovery, particularly in the first stages of gut healing.

A diverse, nutrient-dense diet helps close repletion gaps and maintain remission.

While convenient, processed gluten-free products should complement—not replace—whole food choices.

True recovery involves more than gluten removal; it requires intentional nourishment and gut support.

Sustained digestive function and optimal long-term outcomes rely on individualized care, balanced nutrition, professional oversight, and evidence-based strategies tailored to each person's needs.

Part III:
Gut Repair & Rebuilding

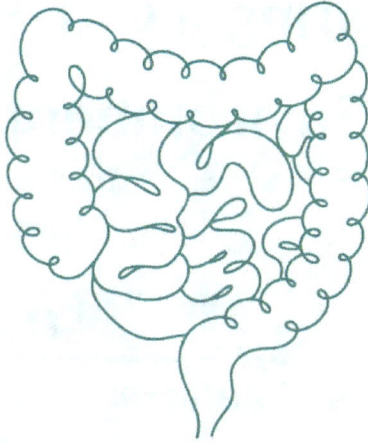

Functional Tools to Restore Balance & Digestive Confidence

Even when gluten is out of the picture, the gut may take months or even years to heal. This section focuses on restoring gut health, regulating symptoms without fear, rebuilding dietary confidence using functional, sustainable strategies.

Chapter 7:
Creating a Gut-Safe Environment

Gut Repair Is Multifactorial: A Whole-Body Approach to Digestive Recovery

Healing the gut—whether from Celiac Disease, IBS, or chronic inflammation—**goes far beyond food alone**. While diet is central, gut health is influenced by a network of systems, including the immune system, nervous system, and hormonal responses. Addressing **all aspects**—nutrition, stress, sleep, and lifestyle—provides the best chance for long-term regulation.

1. Anti-Inflammatory Diets: Fueling the Gut with Nutrient Dense Foods

Certain foods help reduce inflammation and support a more balanced gut microbiome. An **anti-inflammatory diet** rich in plant-based, nutrient-dense ingredients helps reduce immune overactivation in the digestive tract and encourages repair of the gut lining.

- **Omega-3 fatty acids**, found in flaxseeds, walnuts, and fatty fish, — SMASH also known as salmon, mackerel, anchovies, sardines, and herring — a great way to remember the five-cold water fish that are good sources of Omega-3 fatty acids, have been shown to reduce the production of pro-inflammatory cytokines and may improve intestinal barrier function (Calder, 2020). These Omega-3 fatty acids are also linked to improved microbiota diversity and a reduction in systemic inflammation.

- **Polyphenols**, the antioxidant compounds found in berries, olive oil, green tea, and herbs, help regulate gut bacteria and lower inflammation. Polyphenols can act as prebiotics, feeding beneficial bacteria like Lactobacillus and Bifidobacterium (Rodríguez-Daza et al., 2021).

- **High-fiber foods**—especially soluble fibers from oats, legumes, chia seeds, and vegetables—feed gut microbes and support the production of **short-chain fatty acids (SCFAs)**, which help reduce inflammation and protect gut lining integrity (Biesiekierski et al., 2013).

2. Gut Barrier Support: Rebuilding the Intestinal Wall

When the gut is inflamed or damaged, the **tight junctions** between intestinal cells can loosen, allowing unwanted substances to "leak" into the bloodstream—a condition often called "leaky gut" or increased intestinal permeability. Supporting the repair of this barrier is essential.

- **L-glutamine**, an amino acid, serves as a primary fuel source for the cells lining the small intestine. Recent studies suggest glutamine supplementation may help restore barrier function and reduce intestinal permeability, especially in inflammatory bowel conditions ((Freitas et al., 2018)

- **Zinc** supports wound healing and has been shown to regulate tight junction proteins in the gut. It plays a crucial role in mucosal immunity and epithelial regeneration (Wessels et al., 2017). In conditions like Crohn's disease and Celiac Disease, zinc supplementation has been associated with faster mucosal recovery.

- **Resistant starches** (e.g., green bananas, cooked-and-cooled potatoes, legumes) are a type of fermentable fiber that gut bacteria convert into SCFAs—especially **butyrate**, which fuels colon cells and helps reduce inflammation (Biesiekierski et al., 2013).

3. Sleep, Stress & the Gut-Brain Axis: Repair Beyond the Digestive Tract

Communication between the brain and gut occurs constantly through the **gut-brain axis**—a two-way communication system involving nerves, hormones, and immune messengers. Stress and poor sleep can worsen dysbiosis (imbalance in gut bacteria), increase intestinal permeability, and amplify inflammation.

- **Chronic stress** activates the hypothalamic-pituitary-adrenal (HPA) axis, releasing cortisol and other stress hormones that impair digestion and alter the gut microbiota. Chronic stress not only disrupts gut barrier integrity but also reduces levels of beneficial microbes (Zingone et al., 2015).

3. **Sleep deprivation** has been associated with increased intestinal permeability and heightened inflammatory responses. Partial sleep loss can elevate pro-inflammatory cytokines and reduce

microbial diversity, highlighting the connection between sleep quality and gut health. (Benedict et al., 2016).

Restoring circadian rhythm through consistent sleep, practicing stress management (such as deep breathing, mindfulness, or moderate exercise), and engaging in social connection can support both gut and brain function.

The Bottom Line: A Holistic Gut-Healing Framework

The gut takes more than cutting out trigger foods—it requires a full-body approach. Research shows that chronic digestive issues often stem from a mix of dietary, microbial, and lifestyle imbalances (McClave & Omer, 2020; Qiu et al., 2022). A well-rounded gut-healing strategy includes:

- **Nutrition**: Eating a diet rich in anti-inflammatory foods (like leafy greens, berries, and omega-3 fatty acids), soluble fiber, and targeted nutrients supports gut lining repair. For example, L-glutamine is a key amino acid that helps restore intestinal barrier function (Kim and Kim, 2017) while **zinc** plays a vital role in tight junction integrity and immune defense within the gut (Wessels et al., 2017).

- **Microbial Balance**: A diverse, balanced microbiome is essential for digestion, nutrient absorption, and immune health. Feeding the good gut bacteria with resistant starches (from cooled potatoes, green bananas, and lentils) and polyphenols (from foods like blueberries, olive oil, and green tea) helps reduce inflammation and promote microbial diversity (Rodríguez-Daza et al., 2021).

- **Lifestyle**: Chronic stress and poor sleep disrupt the gut-brain axis, increasing intestinal permeability and altering microbiome composition. Evidence shows that managing stress through breathing exercises, physical activity, and consistent sleep patterns can improve digestive symptoms and reduce inflammatory markers (Chong et al., 2019; Tarawneh and Penhos, 2022).

Together, these elements help restore not just digestive health but also whole-body balance—supporting mood, metabolism, and immune function from the inside out.

Key Takeaways

Gut repair involves nutrition, sleep, and stress regulation.

Anti-inflammatory nutrients support mucosal repair.

The gut-brain connection is real—and treatable.

Chapter 8:
Tracking Symptoms
Without Obsession

Symptom Journals: Finding the Balance Between Awareness and Anxiety

For individuals navigating chronic digestive conditions—such as Celiac Disease, IBS, or functional dyspepsia—**symptom tracking** can be a powerful tool. It helps connect patterns between food, mood, bowel habits, and other lifestyle factors. However, **too much tracking** or a hyper-focus on every meal, symptom, or reaction can backfire, leading to **anxiety**, fear of food, and **disordered eating behaviors**.

Why Symptom Tracking Helps (When Used Thoughtfully)

A well-structured food and symptom journal allows individuals to:

- Identify trends over **several days** (rather than obsessing over a single food or symptom)

- Observe how symptoms correlate with **mood, stress, sleep**, and **bowel habits**

- Empower informed discussions with a provider or RDN

- Begin building a sense of **trust and understanding** with their body

Tracking becomes especially helpful in conditions like IBS or CD, where triggers are often multifactorial and not always immediate. Logging the **timing of symptoms** (e.g., 30 minutes vs. 6 hours after eating) can help differentiate between **upper GI vs. lower GI reactions** or distinguish **food intolerance** from **delayed hypersensitivity**.

But There's a Downside: When Tracking Becomes Harmful

If done rigidly or obsessively, tracking can turn into a source of **psychological stress** and may even mimic the behaviors seen in disordered eating.

Individuals with gastrointestinal conditions often experience increased **food-related anxiety**, **fear of eating**, and **emotional distress**, especially when they feel they must constantly monitor symptoms and restrict foods to avoid discomfort. This kind of hypervigilance can create a **cycle of fear and avoidance**, which makes social eating or trying new foods overwhelming (Satherley et al., 2015).

Similarly, in adults with Celiac Disease, over-focusing on food choices—even when medically necessary—can significantly lower **quality of life** and contribute to social isolation or rigid eating behaviors, especially if tracking is tied to perfectionism or fear of symptoms (Al-sunaid et al., 2021).

Excessive monitoring may also contribute to **orthorexic tendencies** (an obsession with "clean" or "safe" eating), particularly when individuals begin to categorize foods as inherently "good" or "bad" based on single reactions rather than patterns.

A Better Approach: Use Symptom Journals as a Tool—Not a Rule

To use symptom tracking in a **constructive, non-anxious way**:

Log more than food: Include timing, mood, bowel habits, energy, sleep, and stress. This gives context to symptoms and widens the lens beyond food alone.

Look for patterns over time: Focus on repeating trends across days or weeks—not isolated events. The body is not a machine; minor fluctuations are normal.

Avoid harsh self-judgment: Tracking is a form of data collection, not a test that is pass or fail. The goal is curiosity, not control.

Working with a provider: Sharing the journal with an RDN or GI specialist can help make sense of confusing trends and prevent unnecessary restriction.

Key Takeaways

Tracking can be empowering when it's used to gather insight—not impose rules.

Focus on patterns, not perfection. The gut is influenced by more than just food—emotions, stress, and hormones all matter too.

Let symptom journals guide understanding, not punishment. Use them to foster trust in the body, not fear of it.

Chapter 9:
Working with an RDN Who Gets It

Why Personalized Nutrition Support Matters for Digestive Health

Digestive issues like Celiac Disease, IBS, SIBO, and food intolerances are **deeply personal and complex**. What triggers symptoms for one person may not be the same in another. That's why generic meal plans or one-size-fits-all diets often fall short. **Personalized care**—led by an RDN with experience in gastrointestinal (GI) disorders—is invaluable in guiding patients to navigate symptoms.

1. Identifying Needs: Nutrient Gaps, Food Triggers, and Lifestyle Obstacles

A GI RDN takes a comprehensive view of an individual's health—going beyond food diaries or symptom lists.

Incorporating:

- **Micronutrient status**: People with chronic GI conditions are more likely to have deficiencies in iron, B12, folate, Vitamin D, zinc, and magnesium due to inflammation or malabsorption. A 2024 retrospective cohort study published in Digestive Diseases and Sciences evaluated the impact of a dedicated Celiac Disease program, which included specialized RDN support, on patients with Celiac Disease. The study found that participants in the program achieved higher adherence to quality care metrics, experienced greater symptom resolution— particularly of gastrointestinal symptoms like diarrhea and bloating—

and demonstrated improved short-term outcomes compared to those receiving standard care. These findings underscore the critical role of multidisciplinary management, including RDN involvement, in enhancing patient outcomes in Celiac Disease (Ford et al., 2024)

- **Food triggers**: Identifying sensitivities can be tricky—especially when symptoms are delayed or inconsistent. Instead of eliminating everything all at once (which can lead to under-eating or nutrient deficiencies), RDN use **targeted, stepwise approaches** to narrow down what's truly causing discomfort.

- **Lifestyle barriers**: Stress, sleep, work schedules, and even cultural eating patterns affect digestion. An RDN helps uncover which habits might be working against an individual and builds realistic strategies that honor their life—not just their lab results.

2. Functional Testing (When It's Clinically Appropriate)

In some cases, an RDN may recommend **functional GI testing** to help clarify root causes—especially when symptoms persist despite dietary changes. These may include:

- **Comprehensive stool analysis** to assess inflammation markers, digestive enzymes, gut bacteria, and pathogens

- **SIBO** breath testing, which measures hydrogen/methane levels produced by bacteria in the small intestine

- **Micronutrient panels** to evaluate stored nutrient levels that might not show up on basic labs

While not always necessary, these tools can give valuable insight when used appropriately as part of a **clinical picture**—not in isolation or for fear-based testing.

Key point: An RDN helps interpret results in a way that leads to clear action—not confusion or unnecessary restriction.

3. Supervised Food Reintroductions (No More Guesswork or Over-Restriction)

A major challenge for many people with GI symptoms is **fear of food, bloating, frequent bathroom visits**, and **flare-ups**. As a result, many people start to eliminate more and more foods, which can lead to a restricted diet, nutrient deficiencies, and even social withdrawal.

This is where **supervised reintroduction trials** come in.

Under the guidance of an RDN, foods are slowly reintroduced in a **structured**, **supportive**, and **evidence-based manner** to assess tolerance. These trials:

- Help rebuild confidence around food
- Clarify true triggers vs. unnecessary restrictions
- Restore variety, flexibility, and enjoyment to eating

- Prevent the nutritional and psychological consequences of long-term avoidance

RDNs are uniquely equipped to oversee the reintroduction of foods in individuals with Celiac Disease and related gastrointestinal conditions. Specialized training spans both the biological mechanisms of food sensitivities with the psychological aspects of eating behaviors—domains that are often underrepresented in primary care. This dual expertise allows RDNs to tailor nutrition interventions that address both physiological tolerance and emotional readiness, fostering more sustainable and patient-centered outcomes (McDermid et al., 2023).

4. Behavioral and Emotional Support

Chronic digestive conditions don't just affect the gut—they impact **how people think and feel about food**. Many patients report anxiety before meals, confusion over symptoms, and feeling like food is the enemy. As an RDN:

- Reframe negative food experiences and reduce food fear
- Set realistic, sustainable goals—not perfection
- Navigate social eating, travel, and life transitions with confidence
- Build a flexible, compassionate relationship with food

This support is not "just emotional"—it's **evidence-based behavioral counseling** that supports long-term health outcomes and quality of life.

Key Takeaways

Personalized care helps to stop guessing and start healing

RDNs translate labs, patterns, and symptoms into clear, safe action steps

Use of evidence-based guidance that respects each unique story, culture, and experiences

Digestive healing is not about restriction—it's about reconnection. Professional support can move beyond symptom-chasing and aid individuals to be confident in their food choices again.

Part IV:
Long-Term Repair
and Emotional Resilience

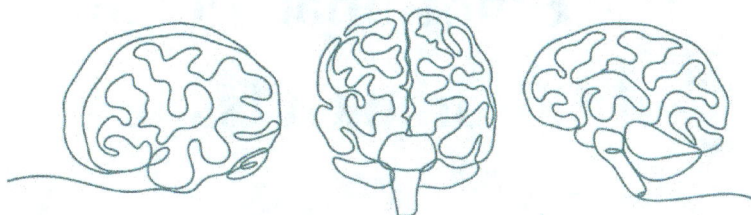

From Food Fear to Freedom—Restoring Joy, Identity, and Confidence

Living with Celiac Disease or ongoing digestive symptoms often extends beyond food. It affects social lives, mental health, relationships, and self-image. This section offers strategies to reclaim a balanced relationship with food, rebuild trust, and define long-term health beyond symptom management.

Chapter 10:
The Emotional Weight
of Chronic GI Issues

When the Gut Hurts, the Mind Hurts Too: Understanding the Emotional Impact of Celiac Disease and IBS

Living with a chronic digestive condition like **Celiac Disease** or **IBS** doesn't just affect the gut—it affects the whole person. Research shows that people with these conditions are at a significantly higher risk for **anxiety**, **depression**, and **social withdrawal**, especially when symptoms persist despite their best efforts to eat "correctly" or follow strict diets (Zingone et al., 2015).

This isn't a sign of weakness or failure—**it's a common and valid part of the experience**.

Gut disorders and mental health are deeply connected through the **gut-brain axis**—a two-way communication system between the digestive system and the brain. When the gut is inflamed, unbalanced, or under distress, it sends signals to the brain that can affect mood, clarity, and emotional regulation.

Why Digestive Disorders Affect Mental Health

Multiple studies show that people with Celiac Disease or IBS are more likely to experience:

- **Anxiety and panic around eating**, especially in social settings

- **Fear of cross-contamination**, especially with gluten-containing foods

- **Shame or frustration** from unpredictable symptoms

- **Loss of control** or **identity confusion**, especially when diagnoses are unclear

- **Isolation**, especially when friends and family don't understand dietary needs

Individuals with Celiac Disease—particularly those recently diagnosed or still experiencing symptoms—show significantly higher rates of **generalized anxiety, health-related fears**, and **reduced social engagement**. These issues are particularly heightened in people who have struggled for years without a diagnosis or have had their symptoms dismissed (Zingone et al., 2015).

Similarly, people with IBS often face **increased emotional sensitivity** due to changes in serotonin signaling within the gut. Serotonin, commonly known as the "feel-good" chemical, is produced in large amounts in the gut, and disturbances in gut health can reduce its effectiveness, contributing to **low mood, irritability**, and **depressive symptoms** (Almazar et al., 2018).

How Emotional Distress Can Impact Eating Patterns

When managing symptoms becomes a daily battle, it's understandable that food begins to feel like a threat rather than nourishment. Over time, this can lead to **disordered eating behaviors**, such as:

- **Orthorexia** – An unhealthy fixation on eating only "pure" or "safe" foods, often leading to excessive restriction

- **Avoidant/Restrictive Food Intake Disorder (ARFID)** – Avoidance of food due to fear of symptoms or past traumatic eating experiences

- **Emotional eating** or **stress avoidance of food altogether** due to digestive flare-ups or past negative experiences with food

These behaviors can worsen nutritional status, disrupt social connection, and even increase the risk of malnutrition—despite being rooted in the goal of **feeling better**.

Mental Health Support Is Essential—Not Optional

Mental health matters just as much as physical gut symptoms. Emotional distress around food isn't just a side effect of digestive disease—it's a part of the disease burden itself.

The **good news** is that mental and physical symptoms can improve with the right support:

- **RDNs** trained in GI disorders can help reduce food fear and rebuild confidence with structured reintroductions and flexible meal planning

- **Mental health providers**, particularly those familiar with chronic illness or eating disorders, can help address trauma, anxiety, and body trust issues

- **GI specialists** ensure accurate diagnosis and rule out medical causes of symptoms

Key Takeaways

Mental health is inseparable from gut health—the brain and the gut are in constant conversation.

Emotional distress often comes from fear and uncertainty, not personal failure.

A multidisciplinary care team—including an RDN, GI provider, and therapist—offers the most effective and compassionate support.

Chapter 11:
Redefining "Healthy"

Beyond Food Rules: Redefining What It Means to Be "Healthy" with a Chronic GI Condition

Individuals living with a digestive disorder like **Celiac Disease, IBS, SIBO**, or **food intolerances**, encounter an overwhelming number of "wellness rules":

Gluten-free. Dairy-free. Low-FODMAP. No sugar. No carbs. No fun.

While some of these approaches are medically necessary or temporarily helpful, **a life of permanent restriction isn't the goal—it's a detour on the path to sustainable, joyful nourishment**.

Real health isn't built on rules—it's built on flexibility, function, and self-trust.

Moving Away from Food Fear Toward

Food Freedom

Instead of focusing on strict rules, recent research supports an approach that builds **a balanced relationship with food**, particularly in people with chronic GI symptoms. This includes:

Instead of:	Try this:
Calorie counting	Visual guides for portion balance
Eliminating every trigger	Strategic reintroduction with support
Obsessive food tracking	Pattern awareness across meals and moods
Following rigid food lists	Flexible food frameworks tailored to an individual

This doesn't mean ignoring symptoms or abandoning structure—it means creating a more **sustainable, kind**, and **body-aware** approach to managing them.

What the Research Says About Flexible, Whole-Person Approaches

Intuitive eating—an approach that focuses on hunger cues, satisfaction, and body respect—is associated with **lower rates of disordered eating, higher psychological well-being**, and **improved self-esteem**, without compromising physical health outcomes (Babbott et al., 2023).

This is especially important for people with GI disorders who may feel **pressured to micromanage their diets** or avoid social situations due to food anxiety. The review highlights how intuitive eating can **coexist with necessary medical diets**, when framed through the lens of **flexibility** and **self-awareness** rather than rigidity and fear.

Additionally, individuals with IBS, **perceived stigma** and **emotional distress** often had a stronger impact on quality of life than physical symptoms themselves. When patients felt unsupported, ashamed, or judged for their condition, they were more likely to develop maladaptive eating behaviors and social withdrawal. In contrast, **compassionate, person-centered care** improved both symptom coping and emotional resilience (Dakó et al., 2024).

Core Concepts in HAES-Informed and Intuitive Eating Care

- **Body Trust**: Learning to listen to the body's cues, not just follow external rules. This includes honoring hunger, fullness, and even cravings with curiosity rather than judgment.

- **Functional Eating**: Eating for how food makes an individual feel—not just how it fits into a diet plan. This may include noticing energy, digestion, mood, and mental clarity as a guide.

- **Mental & Emotional Well-being**: Protecting the relationship with food, body, and sense of identity—giving them as much as lab values. Chronic illness isn't just a physical experience—it's deeply emotional too.

This approach can be especially healing for individuals who have spent years fearing food or defining health as the absence of symptoms. It makes space for **joy, culture, spontaneity**, and **dignity**.

Key Takeaways

Health is more than symptom suppression—it includes emotional safety, confidence, and quality of life.

Redefining "healthy" makes room for cultural foods, favorite memories, and shared meals—without shame.

The body is not broken or failing—it can become a partner, not a project.

Conclusion:
Support Beyond
Dietary Elimination

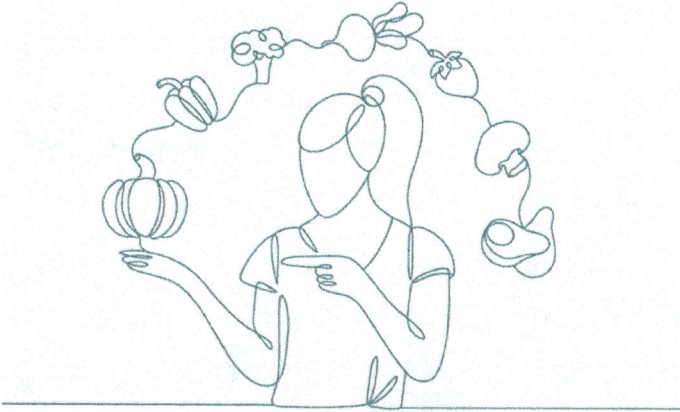

Managing Celiac Disease, IBS, and related GI conditions extends beyond food avoidance—it requires a comprehensive, patient-centered approach.

Many individuals continue to experience symptoms despite dietary adherence or carry uncertain diagnoses that leave them without clarity or direction. As clinicians, we play a critical role in helping patients make sense of their symptoms, identify contributing factors, and implement evidence-based strategies that support both function and quality of life.

This book is designed to move beyond symptom labeling and restrictive protocols. It provides tools to assess nutritional adequacy, address coexisting GI concerns, and support long-term dietary management without unnecessary limitations. While removing gluten or other triggers may be part of the process, the ultimate goal is to empower patients with the knowledge, structure, and professional guidance they need to move forward with greater confidence and improved well-being.

References

Al-sunaid, Fahdah F., Maha M. Al-homidi, Rawan M. Al-qahtani, Reema A. Al-ashwal, Ghada A. Mudhish, Mahitab A. Hanbazaza, and Abeer S. Al-zaben. "The Influence of a Gluten-Free Diet on Health-Related Quality of Life in Individuals with Celiac Disease." BMC Gastroenterology 21 (August 25, 2021): 330. https://doi.org/10.1186/s12876-021-01908-0.

Almazar, Ann E., Nicholas J. Talley, Tricia L. Brantner, Joseph J. Larson, Elizabeth J. Atkinson, Joseph A. Murray, and Yuri A. Saito. "Celiac Disease is Uncommon in Irritable Bowel Syndrome in the United States." European Journal of Gastroenterology & Hepatology 30, no. 2 (February 2018): 149–54. (Freitas et al., 2018).

Armand, Martine. "Lipases and Lipolysis in the Human Digestive Tract: Where Do We Stand?" Current Opinion in Clinical Nutrition and Metabolic Care 10, no. 2 (March 2007): 156–64. https://doi.org/10.1097/MCO.0b013e3280177687.

Babbott, Katie M., Alana Cavadino, Jennifer Brenton-Peters, Nathan S. Consedine, and Marion Roberts. "Outcomes of Intuitive Eating Interventions: A Systematic Review and Meta-Analysis." Eating Disorders 31, no. 1 (2023): 33–63. https://doi.org/10.1080/10640266.2022.2030124.

Basile, Eric J., Marjorie V. Launico, and Amy J. Sheer. "Physiology, Nutrient Absorption." In StatPearls. Treasure Island (FL): StatPearls Publishing, 2025. http://www.ncbi.nlm.nih.gov/books/NBK597379/.

Bellini, Massimo, Sara Tonarelli, Attila G. Nagy, Andrea Pancetti, Francesco Costa, Angelo Ricchiuti, Nicola de Bortoli, Marta Mosca, Santino Marchi, and Alessandra Rossi. "Low FODMAP Diet: Evidence, Doubts, and Hopes." Nutrients 12, no. 1 (January 2020): 148. https://doi.org/10.3390/nu12010148.

Biesiekierski, Jessica R., Simone L. Peters, Evan D. Newnham, Ourania Rosella, Jane G. Muir, and Peter R. Gibson. "No Effects of Gluten in Patients with Self-Reported Non-Celiac Gluten Sensitivity After Dietary Reduction of Fermentable, Poorly Absorbed, Short-Chain Carbohydrates." Gastroenterology 145, no. 2 (August 1, 2013): 320-328.e3. https://doi.org/10.1053/j.gastro.2013.04.051.

Caio, Giacomo, Umberto Volta, Anna Sapone, Daniel A. Leffler, Roberto De Giorgio, Carlo Catassi, and Alessio Fasano. "Celiac Disease: A Comprehensive Current Review." BMC Medicine 17, no. 1 (July 23, 2019): 142. https://doi.org/10.1186/s12916-019-1380-z.

Chong, Pei Pei, Voon Kin Chin, Chung Yeng Looi, Won Fen Wong, Priya Madhavan, and Voon Chen Yong. "The Microbiome and Irritable Bowel Syndrome - A Review on the Pathophysiology, Current Research and Future Therapy." Frontiers in Microbiology 10 (2019): 1136. https://doi.org/10.3389/fmicb.2019.01136.

Crowell, Michael D. "Role of Serotonin in the Pathophysiology of the Irritable Bowel Syndrome." British Journal of Pharmacology 141, no. 8 (April 2004): 1285–93. https://doi.org/10.1038/sj.bjp.0705762.

Dakó, Eszter, Sarolta Dakó, Veronika Papp, Márk Juhász, Johanna Takács, Éva Csajbókné Csobod, and Erzsébet Pálfi. "Monitoring the Quality of Life and the Relationship between Quality of Life, Dietary Intervention, and Dietary Adherence in Patients with Coeliac Disease." Nutrients 16, no. 17 (September 3, 2024): 2964. https://doi.org/10.3390/nu16172964.

Di Sabatino, Antonio, and Gino Roberto Corazza. "Coeliac Disease." Lancet (London, England) 373, no. 9673 (April 25, 2009): 1480–93. https://doi.org/10.1016/S0140-6736(09)60254-3.

Freitas, Daniela, Steven Le Feunteun, Maud Panouillé, and Isabelle Souchon. "The Important Role of Salivary ?-Amylase in the Gastric Digestion of Wheat Bread Starch." Food & Function 9, no. 1 (January 24, 2018): 200–208. https://doi.org/10.1039/c7fo01484h.

Gibson, Peter R., Emma P. Halmos, Daniel So, Chu K. Yao, Jane E. Varney, and Jane G. Muir. "Diet as a Therapeutic Tool in Chronic Gastrointestinal Disorders: Lessons from the FODMAP Journey." Journal of Gastroenterology and Hepatology 37, no. 4 (April 2022): 644–52. https://doi.org/10.1111/jgh.15772.

Green, Peter H. R., and Christophe Cellier. "Celiac Disease." The New England Journal of Medicine 357, no. 17 (October 25, 2007): 1731–43. https://doi.org/10.1056/NEJMra071600.

Hallert, C., C. Grant, S. Grehn, C. Grännö, S. Hultén, G. Midhagen, M. Ström, H. Svensson, and T. Valdimarsson. "Evidence of Poor Vitamin Status in Coeliac Patients on a Gluten-Free Diet for 10 Years." Alimentary Pharmacology & Therapeutics 16, no. 7 (July 2002): 1333–39. https://doi.org/10.1046/j.1365-2036.2002.01283.x.

Hill, Ivor D., Alessio Fasano, Stefano Guandalini, Edward Hoffenberg, Joseph Levy, Norelle Reilly, and Ritu Verma. "NASPGHAN Clinical Report on the Diagnosis and Treatment of Gluten-Related Disorders." Journal of Pediatric Gastroenterology and Nutrition 63, no. 1 (July 2016): 156–65. https://doi.org/10.1097/MPG.0000000000001216.

Husby, Steffen, Sibylle Koletzko, Ilma Korponay-Szabó, Kalle Kurppa, Maria Luisa Mearin, Carmen Ribes-Koninckx, Raanan Shamir, et al. "European Society Paediatric Gastroenterology, Hepatology and Nutrition Guidelines for Diagnosing Coeliac Disease 2020." Journal of Pediatric Gastroenterology and Nutrition 70, no. 1 (January 2020): 141–56. https://doi.org/10.1097/MPG.0000000000002497.

Kim, Min-Hyun, and Hyeyoung Kim. "The Roles of Glutamine in the Intestine and Its Implication in Intestinal Diseases." International Journal of Molecular Sciences 18, no. 5 (May 12, 2017): 1051. https://doi.org/10.3390/ijms18051051.

Lebwohl, Benjamin, Alberto Rubio-Tapia, Asaad Assiri, Catherine Newland, and Stefano Guandalini. "Diagnosis of Celiac Disease." Gastrointestinal Endoscopy Clinics of North America 22, no. 4 (October 2012): 661–77. https://doi.org/10.1016/j.giec.2012.07.004.

Leonard, Maureen M., Jocelyn A. Silvester, Daniel Leffler, Alessio Fasano, Ciarán P. Kelly, Suzanne K. Lewis, Jeffrey D. Goldsmith, et al. "Evaluating Responses to Gluten Challenge: A Randomized, Double-Blind, 2-Dose Gluten Challenge Trial." Gastroenterology 160, no. 3 (February 2021): 720-733.e8. https://doi.org/10.1053/j.gastro.2020.10.040.

McClave, Stephen A., and Endashaw Omer. "Clinical Nutrition for the Gastroenterologist: Bedside Strategies for Feeding the Hospitalized Patient." Current Opinion in Gastroenterology 36, no. 2 (March 2020): 122. https://doi.org/10.1097/MOG.0000000000000617.

McGill, Sarah K., Roy Soetikno, Robert V. Rouse, Hobart Lai, and Tonya Kaltenbach. "Patients With Nonpolypoid (Flat and Depressed) Colorectal Neoplasms at Increased Risk for Advanced Neoplasias, Compared with Patients with Polypoid Neoplasms." Clinical Gastroenterology and Hepatology 15, no. 2 (February 1, 2017): 249-256.e1. https://doi.org/10.1016/j.cgh.2016.08.045.

McLean, Thomas C., Rebecca Lo, Natalia Tschowri, Paul A. Hoskisson, Mahmoud M. Al Bassam, Matthew I. Hutchings, and Nicolle F. Som. "Sensing and Responding to Diverse Extracellular Signals: An Updated Analysis of the Sensor Kinases and Response Regulators of Streptomyces Species | Microbiology Society." (January 3, 2025): https://www.microbiologyresearch.org/content/journal/micro/10.1099/mic.0.000817.

Missbach, Benjamin, Lukas Schwingshackl, Alina Billmann, Aleksandra Mystek, Melanie Hickelsberger, Gregor Bauer, and Jürgen König. "Gluten-Free Food Database: The Nutritional Quality and Cost of Packaged Gluten-Free Foods." PeerJ 3 (2015): e1337. https://doi.org/10.7717/peerj.1337.

Pinto-Sanchez, M. Ines, Jedid-Jah Blom, Peter R. Gibson, and David Armstrong. "Nutrition Assessment and Management in Celiac Disease." Gastroenterology 167, no. 1 (June 2024): 116-131.e1. https://doi.org/10.1053/j.gastro.2024.02.049.

Qiu, Peng, Takatsugu Ishimoto, Lingfeng Fu, Jun Zhang, Zhenyong Zhang, and Yang Liu. "The Gut Microbiota in Inflammatory Bowel Disease." Frontiers in Cellular and Infection Microbiology 12 (February 22, 2022). https://doi.org/10.3389/fcimb.2022.733992.

Rodríguez-Daza, Maria Carolina, Elena C. Pulido-Mateos, Joseph Lupien-Meilleur, Denis Guyonnet, Yves Desjardins, and Denis Roy. "Polyphenol-Mediated Gut Microbiota Modulation: Toward Prebiotics and Further." Frontiers in Nutrition 8 (June 28, 2021): 689456. https://doi.org/10.3389/fnut.2021.689456.

Roos, Susanne, Gunilla M. Liedberg, Ingrid Hellström, and Susan Wilhelmsson. "Persistent Symptoms in People with Celiac Disease Despite Gluten-Free Diet: A Concern?" Gastroenterology Nursing: The Official Journal of the Society of Gastroenterology Nurses and Associates 42, no. 6 (2019): 496–503. https://doi.org/10.1097/SGA.0000000000000377.

Rubio-Tapia, Alberto, Ivor D. Hill, Ciarán P.
Kelly, Audrey H. Calderwood, Joseph A.
Murray, and American College of
Gastroenterology. "ACG Clinical Guidelines:
Diagnosis and Management of Celiac
Disease." The American Journal of
Gastroenterology 108, no. 5 (May 2013): 656–
76; quiz 677.
https://doi.org/10.1038/ajg.2013.79.

Ryan, B. M., and D. Kelleher. "Refractory Celiac
Disease." Gastroenterology 119, no. 1 (July
2000): 243–51.
https://doi.org/10.1053/gast.2000.8530.

Satherley, R., R. Howard, and S. Higgs.
"Disordered Eating Practices in
Gastrointestinal Disorders." Appetite 84
(January 2015): 240–50.
https://doi.org/10.1016/j.appet.2014.10.006.

Shahbazkhani, B., M. Forootan, S. Merat, M. R.
Akbari, S. Nasserimoghadam, H. Vahedi, and
R. Malekzadeh. "Coeliac Disease Presenting
with Symptoms of Irritable Bowel Syndrome."
Alimentary Pharmacology & Therapeutics 18,
no. 2 (July 15, 2003): 231–35.
https://doi.org/10.1046/j.1365-
2036.2003.01666.x.

Shepherd, S. J., and P. R. Gibson. "Nutritional
Inadequacies of the Gluten-Free Diet in Both
Recently-Diagnosed and Long-Term Patients
with Coeliac Disease." Journal of Human
Nutrition and Dietetics: The Official Journal
of the British Dietetic Association 26, no. 4
(August 2013): 349–58.
https://doi.org/10.1111/jhn.12018.

Silvester, Jocelyn A., Isabel Comino, Ciarán P. Kelly, Carolina Sousa, Donald R. Duerksen, and DOGGIE BAG Study Group. "Most Patients with Celiac Disease on Gluten-Free Diets Consume Measurable Amounts of Gluten." Gastroenterology 158, no. 5 (April 2020): 1497-1499.e1. https://doi.org/10.1053/j.gastro.2019.12.016.

Tarawneh, Rawan, and Elena Penhos. "The Gut Microbiome and Alzheimer's Disease: Complex and Bidirectional Interactions." Neuroscience and Biobehavioral Reviews 141 (October 2022): 104814. https://doi.org/10.1016/j.neubiorev.2022.1048 14.

Wessels, Inga, Martina Maywald, and Lothar Rink. "Zinc as a Gatekeeper of Immune Function." Nutrients 9, no. 12 (November 25, 2017): 1286. https://doi.org/10.3390/nu9121286.

Wierdsma, Nicolette J., Marian A. E. van Bokhorst-de van der Schueren, Marijke Berkenpas, Chris J. J. Mulder, and Ad A. van Bodegraven. "Vitamin and Mineral Deficiencies Are Highly Prevalent in Newly Diagnosed Celiac Disease Patients." Nutrients 5, no. 10 (September 30, 2013): 3975–92. https://doi.org/10.3390/nu5103975.

Zingone, Fabiana, Gillian L. Swift, Timothy R.
  Card, David S. Sanders, Jonas F. Ludvigsson,
  and Julio C. Bai. "Psychological Morbidity of
  Celiac Disease: A Review of the Literature."
  United European Gastroenterology Journal 3,
  no. 2 (April 2015): 136–45.
  https://doi.org/10.1177/2050640614560786.

Artwork Small Intestine:

https://depositphotos.com/portfolio-1067125

Artwork Human Digestion System:

https://depositphotos.com/portfolio-5775856

Artwork All other line art:

https://depositphotos.com/portfolio-44775794

About the Author

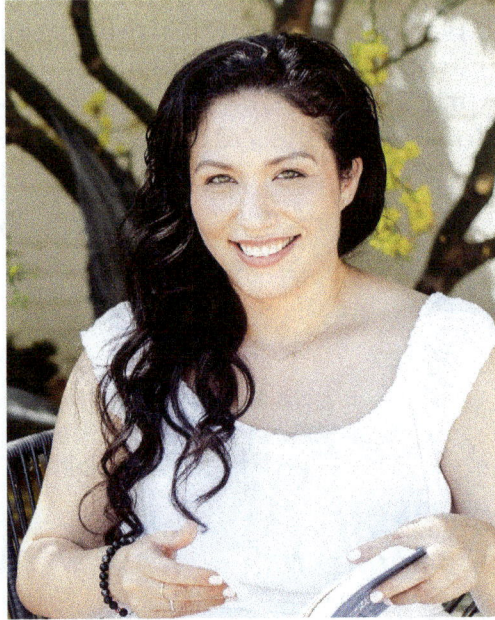

Jessica Martinez, RDN, understands how overwhelming and frustrating the search for answers can be—especially when symptoms persist despite every effort. After nearly a decade of misdiagnoses and being told it was "just IBS," she was finally diagnosed with Celiac Disease in 2015. That experience ignited her commitment to helping others uncover the root causes of chronic digestive issues. A graduate of the Coordinated

Program in Nutrition and Dietetics at Loma Linda University, she brings both clinical expertise and lived experience to her work. She practices in diverse healthcare settings, including hospitals, skilled nursing facilities (SNFs), long-term care (LTC), and private practice.

Behind the Diet: Integrative Nutrition Strategies for Celiac Disease, IBS, and Functional Gut Conditions bridges personal experience with clinical insight to help better recognize and support individuals struggling with chronic gastrointestinal symptoms. Rather than focusing solely on food restrictions, this book explores the systemic patterns, frequent misdiagnoses, and overlooked contributors common in GI conditions. *Behind the Diet* offers a structured, evidence-based framework for identifying red flags, guiding assessments, and improving outcomes through a more integrative lens.

www.ingramcontent.com/pod-product-compliance
Lightning Source LLC
Chambersburg PA
CBHW070924270326
41927CB00011B/2707